The Affordable Cooking

Cheap and Healthy Alkaline Recipes to Save Your Money and Manage Your Weight

Carey Sims

Table of Contents

Most Acid	Acid	Lowest Acid	FOOD CATEGORY	Lowest Alkaline	Alkaline	Most Alkaline
NutraSweet, Equal, Aspartame, Sweet 'N Low	White Sugar, Brown Sugar	Processed Honey, Molasses	SWEETENERS	Raw Honey, Raw Sugar	Maple Syrup, Rice Syrup	Stevia
Blueberries, Cranberries, Prunes	Sour Cherries, Rhubarb	Plums, Processed Fruit Juices	FRUITS	Oranges, Bananas, Cherries, Pineapple, Peaches, Avocados	Dates, Figs, Melons, Grapes, Papaya, Kiwi, Berries, Apples, Pears, Raisins	Lemons, Watermelon, Limes, Grapefruit, Mangoes, Papayas
Chocolate	Potatoes (without skins), Pinto Beans, Navy Beans, Lima Beans	Cooked Spinach, Kidney Beans, String Beans	BEANS VEGETABLES LEGUMES	Carrots, Tomatoes, Fresh Corn, Mushrooms, Cabbage, Peas, Potato Skins, Olives, Soybeans, Tofu	Okra, Squash, Green Beans, Beets, Celery, Lettuce, Zucchini, Sweet Potato, Carob	Asparagus, Onions, Vegetable Juices, Parsley, Raw Spinach, Broccoli, Garlic
Peanuts, Walnuts	Pecans, Cashews	Pumpkin Seeds, Sunflower Seeds	NUTS SEEDS	Chestnuts	Almonds	
		Corn Oil	OILS	Canola Oil	Flax Seed Oil	Olive Oil
Wheat, White Flour, Pastries, Pasta	White Rice, Corn, Buckwheat, Oats, Rye	Sprouted Wheat Bread, Spelt, Brown Rice	GRAINS CEREALS	Amaranth, Millet, Wild Rice, Quinoa		
Beef, Pork, Shellfish	Turkey, Chicken, Lamb	Venison, Cold Water Fish	MEATS			
Cheese, Homogenized Milk, Ice Cream	Raw Milk	Eggs, Butter, Yogurt, Buttermilk, Cottage Cheese	EGGS DAIRY	Soy Cheese, Soy Milk, Goat Milk, Goat Cheese, Whey	Breast Milk	
Beer, Soft Drinks	Coffee	Tea	BEVERAGES	Ginger Tea	Green Tea	Herb Teas, Lemon Water

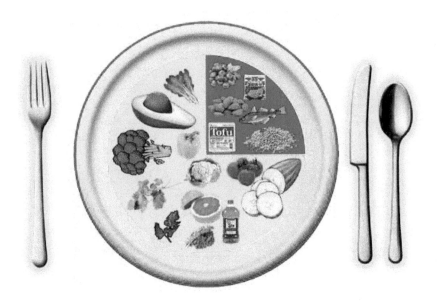

BROCCOLI OMELETTE

Serves: *1*

Prep Time: *5* Minutes

Cook Time: *10* Minutes

Total Time: *15* Minutes

INGREDIENTS

- 2 eggs

- ¼ tsp salt

- ¼ tsp black pepper

- 1 tablespoon olive oil

- ¼ cup cheese

- ¼ tsp basil

- 1 cup broccoli

DIRECTIONS

1. In a bowl combine all ingredients together and mix well

2. In a skillet heat olive oil and pour the egg mixture

3. Cook for 1-2 minutes per side

4. When ready remove omelette from the skillet and serve

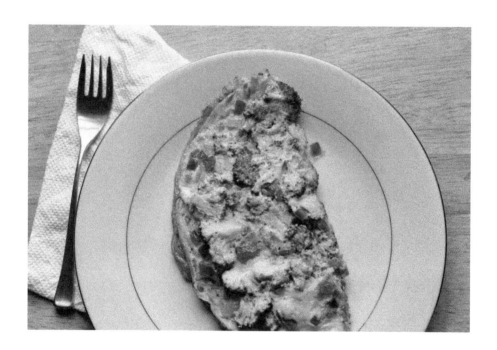

BEETS OMELETTE

Serves: *1*

Prep Time: *5* Minutes

Cook Time: *10* Minutes

Total Time: *15* Minutes

INGREDIENTS

- 2 eggs

- ¼ tsp salt

- ¼ tsp black pepper

- 1 tablespoon olive oil

- ¼ cup cheese

- ¼ tsp basil

- 1 cup beets

DIRECTIONS

1. In a bowl combine all ingredients together and mix well

2. In a skillet heat olive oil and pour the egg mixture

3. Cook for 1-2 minutes per side

4. When ready remove omelette from the skillet and serve

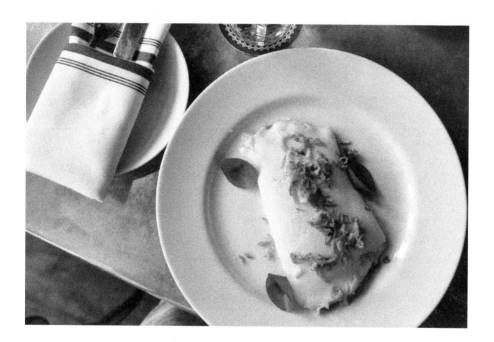

EGGPLANT ROLLATINI

Serves: 6-8

Prep Time: 10 Minutes

Cook Time: 25 Minutes

Total Time: 35 Minutes

INGREDIENTS

- 1 eggplant

- 12 oz. ricotta cheese

- 2 oz. mozzarella cheese

- 1 can tomatoes

- ¼ tsp salt

- 2 tablespoons seasoning

DIRECTIONS

1. Lay the eggplant on a baking sheet

2. Roast at 350 F for 12-15 minutes

3. In a bowl combine mozzarella, seasoning, tomatoes, ricotta cheese and salt

4. Add cheese mixture to the eggplant and roll

5. Place the rolls into a baking dish and bake for another 10-12 minutes

6. When ready remove from the oven and serve

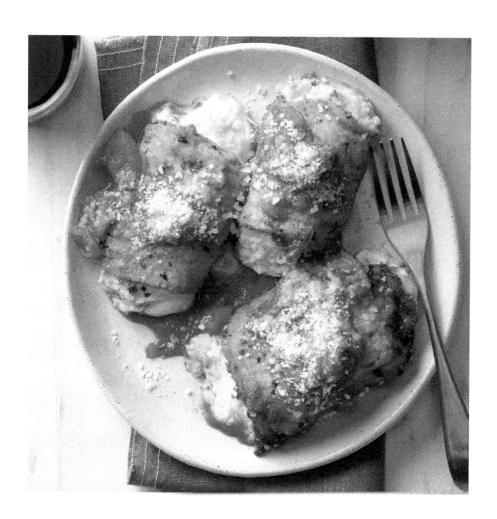

ASPARAGUS WITH EGG

Serves: *4-6*

Prep Time: *10* Minutes

Cook Time: *25* Minutes

Total Time: *35* Minutes

INGREDIENTS

- 1 lb. asparagus

- 4-5 pieces prosciutto

- ¼ tsp salt

- 2 eggs

DIRECTIONS

1. Trim the asparagus and season with salt

2. Wrap each asparagus pieces with prosciutto

3. Place the wrapped asparagus in a baking dish

4. Bake at 375 F for 22-25 minutes

5. When ready remove from the oven and serve

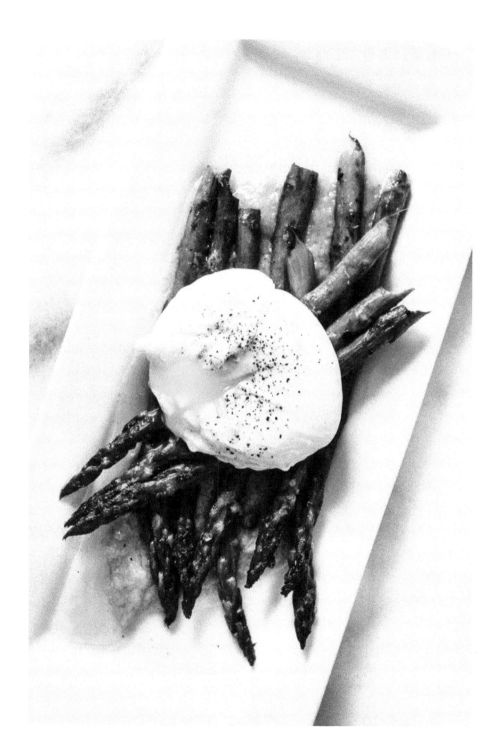

DEVILED EGGS

Serves: 8

Prep Time: 10   Minutes

Cook Time: 20   Minutes

Total Time: 30   Minutes

INGREDIENTS

- 8 eggs

- ½ cup Greek Yogurt

- 1 tablespoon mustard

- 1 tsp smoked paprika

- 1 tablespoon green onions

DIRECTIONS

1. In a saucepan add the eggs and bring to a boil

2. Cover and boil for 10-15 minutes

3. When ready slice the eggs in half and remove the yolks

4. In a bowl combine remaining ingredients and mix well

5. Spoon 1 tablespoon of the mixture into each egg

6. Garnish with green onions and serve

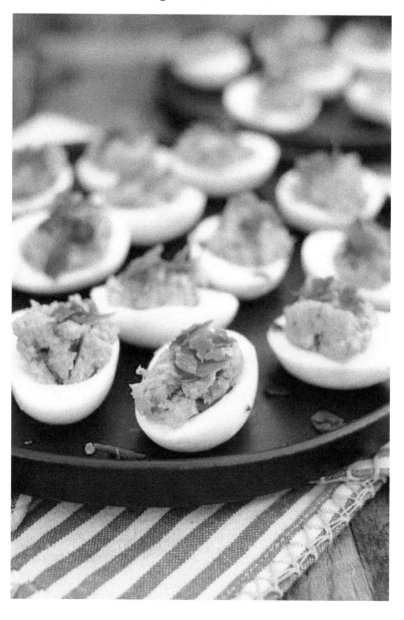

LEEK FRITATTA

Serves: *2*

Prep Time: *10* Minutes

Cook Time: *20* Minutes

Total Time: *30* Minutes

INGREDIENTS

- ½ lb. leek

- 1 tablespoon olive oil

- ½ red onion

- ¼ tsp salt

- 2 ggs

- 2 oz. cheddar cheese

- 1 garlic clove

- ¼ tsp dill

DIRECTIONS

1. In a bowl whisk eggs with salt and cheese

2. In a frying pan heat olive oil and pour egg mixture

3. Add remaining ingredients and mix well

4. Serve when ready

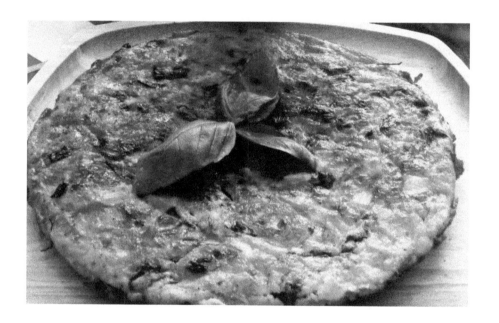

KALE FRITATTA

Serves: *2*

Prep Time: *10* Minutes

Cook Time: *20* Minutes

Total Time: *30* Minutes

INGREDIENTS

- 1 cup kale

- 1 tablespoon olive oil

- ½ red onion

- ¼ tsp salt

- 2 eggs

- 2 oz. cheddar cheese

- 1 garlic clove

- ¼ tsp dill

DIRECTIONS

1. In a skillet sauté kale until tender

2. In a bowl whisk eggs with salt and cheese

3. In a frying pan heat olive oil and pour egg mixture

4. Add remaining ingredients and mix well

5. Serve when ready

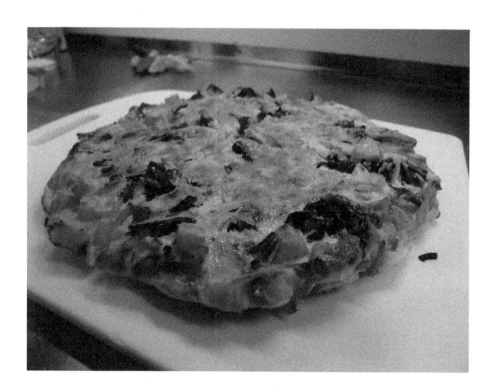

GREENS FRITATTA

Serves: *2*

Prep Time: *10* Minutes

Cook Time: *20* Minutes

Total Time: *30* Minutes

INGREDIENTS

- ½ lb. greens

- 1 tablespoon olive oil

- ½ red onion

- ¼ tsp salt

- 2 eggs

- 2 oz. parmesan cheese

- 1 garlic clove

- ¼ tsp dill

DIRECTIONS

1. In a bowl whisk eggs with salt and parmesan cheese

2. In a frying pan heat olive oil and pour egg mixture

3. Add remaining ingredients and mix well

4. Serve when ready

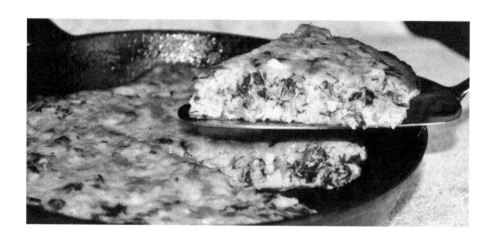

AVOCADO TOAST

Serves: 2

Prep Time: 5   Minutes

Cook Time: 5   Minutes

Total Time: 10   Minutes

INGREDIENTS

- 4 slices bread

- 1 avocado

- ¼ tsp red chili flakes

- ¼ tsp salt

DIRECTIONS

1. Toast the bread and set aside

2. Lay avocado slices on each bread slice

3. Sprinkle with red chili flakes and salt

4. Serve when ready

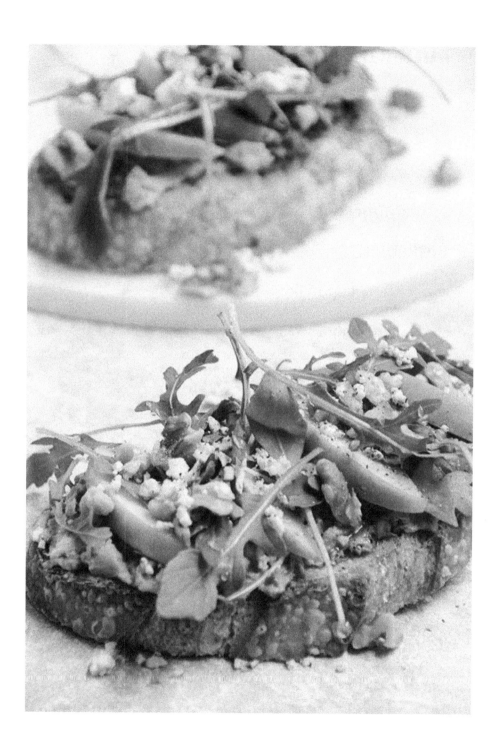

PUMPKIN FRENCH TOAST

Serves: 3

Prep Time: 5 Minutes

Cook Time: 15 Minutes

Total Time: 20 Minutes

INGREDIENTS

- ¼ cup milk

- 2 eggs

- ½ cup pumpkin puree

- 1 tablespoon pumpkin slice

- 6 bread slices

DIRECTIONS

1. In a bowl whisk all ingredients for the dipping

2. Dip the bread into the dipping and let it soak for 3-4 minutes

3. In a skillet heat olive oil and fry each slice for 2-3 minutes per side

4. When ready remove from the skillet and serve

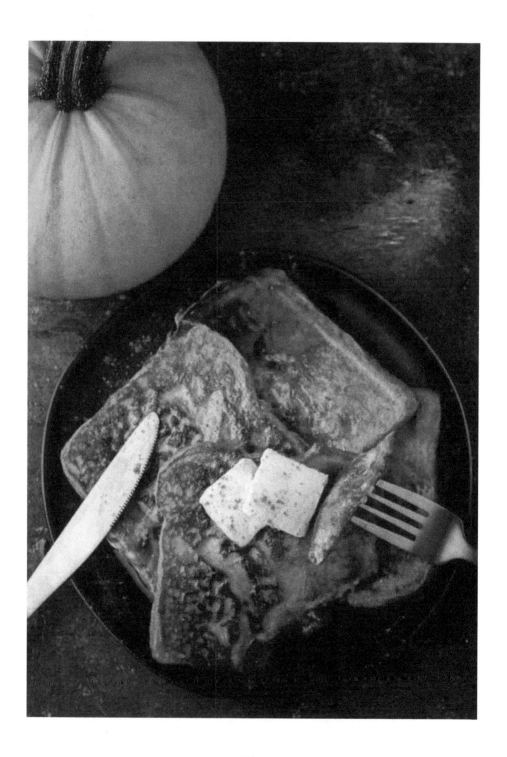

COCONUT CHAI OATMEAL

Serves: 2

Prep Time: 5   Minutes

Cook Time: 15   Minutes

Total Time: 20   Minutes

INGREDIENTS

-        ¼ cup oats

-        ½ cup chia tea

-        ¼ cup coconut milk

-        1 peach

-        ¼ tsp coconut oil

-        1 tsp coconut flakes

DIRECTIONS

1. In a bowl combine together oats, coconut milk, chia tea and microwave until thickness

2. In a saucepan add peach slices and cook for 2-3 minutes

3. Place peaches over the oats and top with coconut flakes

4. Serve when ready

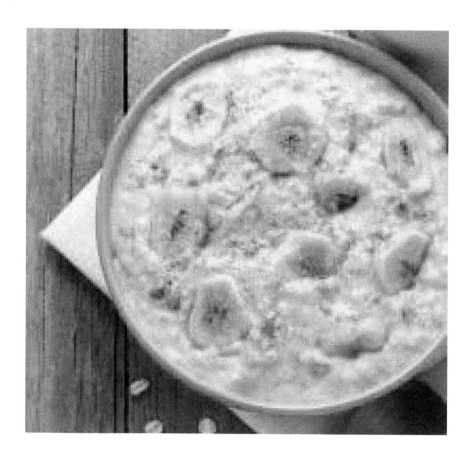

BREAKFAST COOKIES

Serves: 8-12

Prep Time: 5   Minutes

Cook Time: 15   Minutes

Total Time: 20   Minutes

INGREDIENTS

- 1 cup rolled oats

- ¼ cup applesauce

- ½ tsp vanilla extract

- 3 tablespoons chocolate chips

- 2 tablespoons dried fruits

- 1 tsp cinnamon

DIRECTIONS

1. Preheat the oven to 325 F

2. In a bowl combine all ingredients together and mix well

3. Scoop cookies using an ice cream scoop

4. Place cookies onto a prepared baking sheet

5. Place in the oven for 12-15 minutes or until the cookies are done

6. When ready remove from the oven and serve

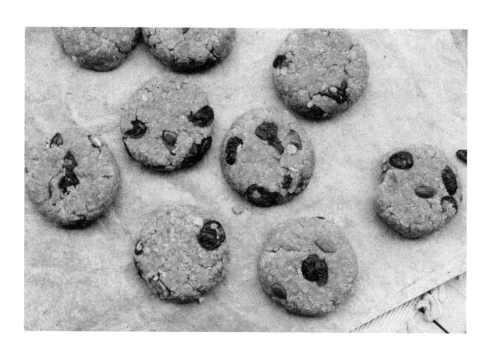

BANANA BREAKFAST SMOOTHIE

Serves: *1*

Prep Time: *5*   Minutes

Cook Time: *5*   Minutes

Total Time: *10*   Minutes

INGREDIENTS

- ½ cup vanilla yogurt

- 2 tsp honey

- Pinch of cinnamon

- 1 banana

- 1 cup ice

DIRECTIONS

1. In a blender place all ingredients and blend until smooth

2. Pour the smoothie in a glass and serve

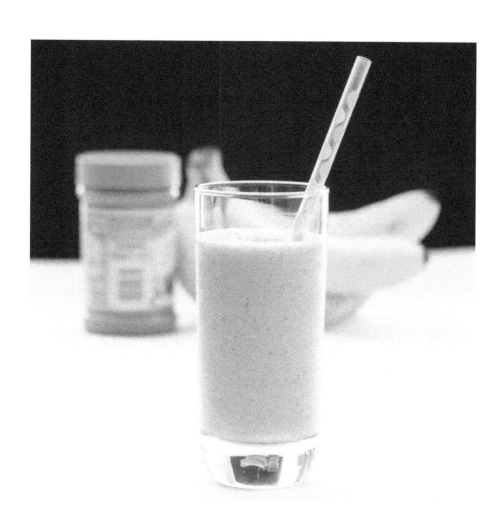

MANGO SMOOTHIE

Serves: *1*

Prep Time: *5*   Minutes

Cook Time: *5*   Minutes

Total Time: *10*   Minutes

INGREDIENTS

-         1 cup coconut milk

-         1 cup vanilla yogurt

-         1 cup ice

-         1 banana

-         1 mango

-         1 tsp vanilla

-         1 tsp honey

DIRECTIONS

1. In a blender place all ingredients and blend until smooth

2. Pour smoothie in a glass and serve

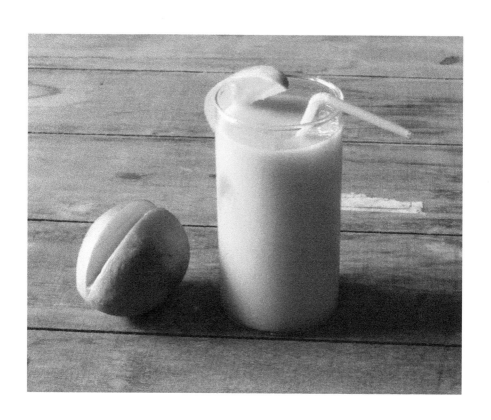

POWER SMOOTHIE

Serves: *1*

Prep Time: *5*   Minutes

Cook Time: *5*   Minutes

Total Time: *10* Minutes

INGREDIENTS

- 2 cups blueberries

- 1 cup pomegranate juice

- 1 cup ice

- 1 tablespoon chia seeds

- 1 banana

DIRECTIONS

1. In a blender place all ingredients and blend until smooth

2. Pour smoothie in a glass and serve

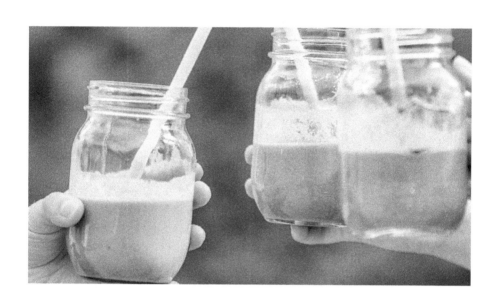

SPINACH SMOOTHIE

Serves: *1*

Prep Time: *5*   Minutes

Cook Time: *5*   Minutes

Total Time: *10*   Minutes

INGREDIENTS

- 1 cup orange juice

- 1 cup coconut water

- 1 banana

- 1 mango

- 2 cups spinach

DIRECTIONS

1. In a blender place all ingredients and blend until smooth

2. Pour smoothie in a glass and serve

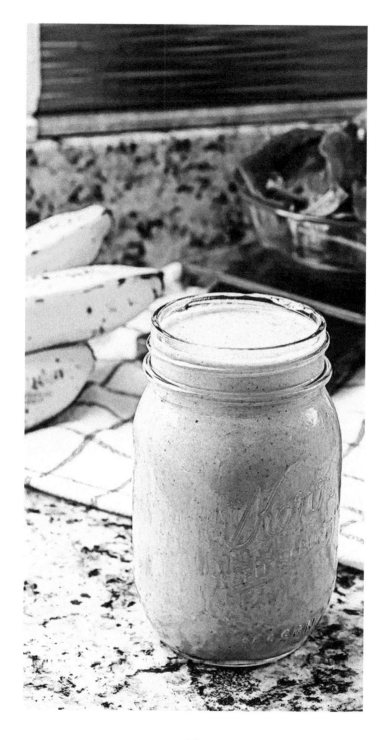

KALE DETOX SMOOTHIE

Serves: *1*

Prep Time: *5*   Minutes

Cook Time: *5*   Minutes

Total Time: *10*   Minutes

INGREDIENTS

-           1 banana

-           1 cup blueberries

-           1 tsp ginger

-           2 cups kale leaves

-           1 cup coconut water

-           1 pinch cinnamon

DIRECTIONS

1. In a blender place all ingredients and blend until smooth

2. Pour smoothie in a glass and serve

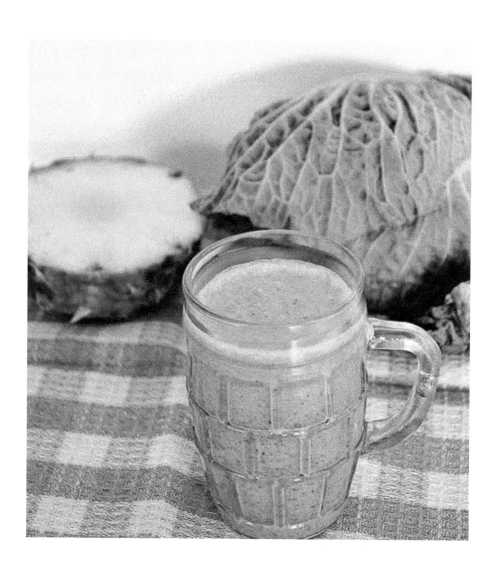

ENERGY BOOSTING SMOOTHIE

Serves: *1*

Prep Time: *5*   Minutes

Cook Time: *5*   Minutes

Total Time: *10* Minutes

INGREDIENTS

-         1 banana

-         1 cup mango

-         1 cup blueberries

-         1 cup Greek Yogurt

-         1 tablespoon honey

-         ¼ avocado

DIRECTIONS

1. In a blender place all ingredients and blend until smooth

2. Pour smoothie in a glass and serve

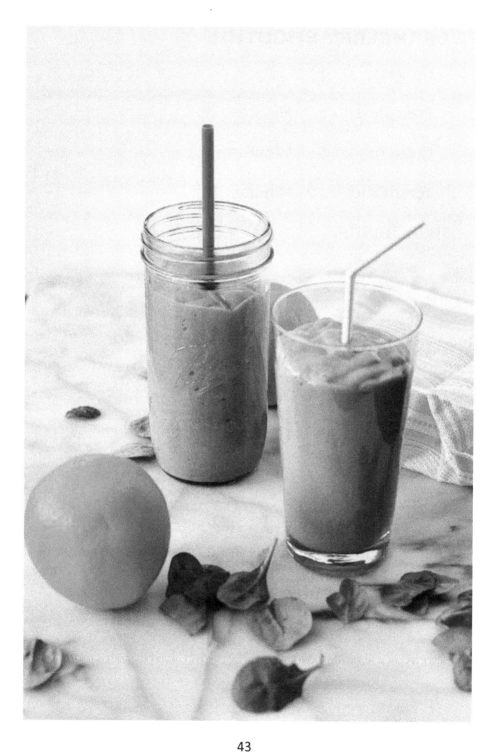

CRANBERRY SMOOTHIE

Serves: *1*

Prep Time: *5*   Minutes

Cook Time: *5*   Minutes

Total Time: *10*   Minutes

INGREDIENTS

- ¼ cup oats

- 1 cup almond milk

- 1 cup cranberry juice

- ¼ cup orange juice

- 1 tablespoon honey

- 1 pinch cinnamon

DIRECTIONS

1. In a blender place all ingredients and blend until smooth

2. Pour smoothie in a glass and serve

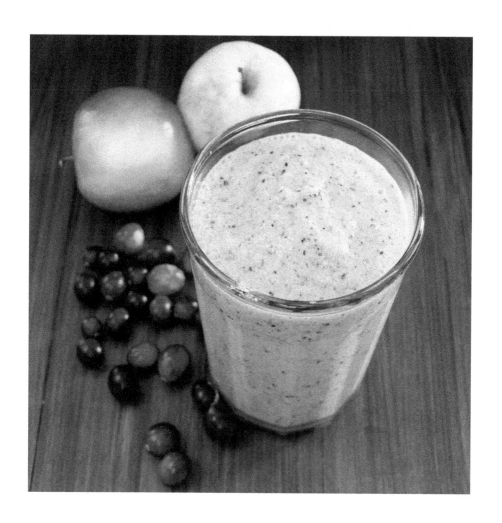

MANDARIN SMOOTHIE

Serves: *1*

Prep Time: *5*   Minutes

Cook Time: *5*   Minutes

Total Time: *10*   Minutes

INGREDIENTS

-        1 cup coconut water

-        1 mandarin orange

-        1 cup frozen blueberries

-        1 tablespoon honey

DIRECTIONS

1. In a blender place all ingredients and blend until smooth

2. Pour smoothie in a glass and serve

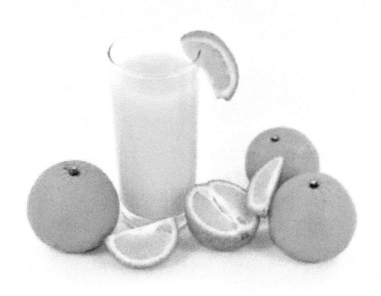

PAPAYA SMOOTHIE

Serves: *1*

Prep Time: *5* Minutes

Cook Time: *5* Minutes

Total Time: *10* Minutes

INGREDIENTS

- 1 banana

- ¼ cup yogurt

- 1 cup papaya

- 1 cup raspberries

- ¼ cup coconut milk

- 1 pinch cinnamon

DIRECTIONS

1. In a blender place all ingredients and blend until smooth

2. Pour smoothie in a glass and serve

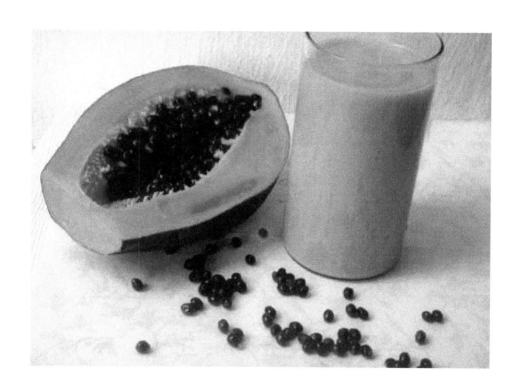

PURPLE SMOOTHIE

Serves: *1*

Prep Time: *5* Minutes

Cook Time: *5* Minutes

Total Time: *10* Minutes

INGREDIENTS

- 1 cup vanilla yogurt

- 1 cup blueberries

- 1 cup blackberries

- 1 cup strawberries

- 1 banana

- 2 tablespoons honey

- 1 cup ice

DIRECTIONS

1. In a blender place all ingredients and blend until smooth

2. Pour smoothie in a glass and serve

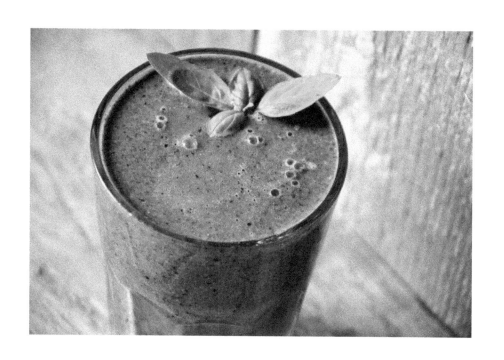

ZUCCHINI SOUP

Serves: *4*

Prep Time: *10* Minutes

Cook Time: *20* Minutes

Total Time: *30* Minutes

INGREDIENTS

- 1 tablespoon olive oil

- 1 lb. zucchini

- ¼ red onion

- ½ cup all-purpose flour

- ¼ tsp salt

- ¼ tsp pepper

- 1 can vegetable broth

- 1 cup heavy cream

DIRECTIONS

1. In a saucepan heat olive oil and sauté zucchini until tender

2. Add remaining ingredients to the saucepan and bring to a boil

3. When all the vegetables are tender transfer to a blender and blend until smooth

4. Pour soup into bowls, garnish with parsley and serve

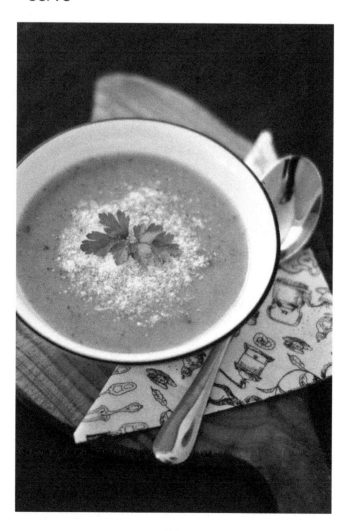

EGGPLANT LENTIL STEW

Serves: *4*

Prep Time: *5* Minutes

Cook Time: *50* Minutes

Total Time: *55* Minutes

INGREDIENTS

- 1 cup lentils

- 2 cups water

- 2 eggplants

- 2 tomatoes

- 2 tablespoons vinegar (SCD safe vinegar)

- 1 tablespoon honey

- 1 tsp basil

- ¼ tsp garlic

- ¼ red pepper flakes

- ¼ tsp onion

DIRECTIONS

1. In a pot bring lentils to a boil, reduce heat and cook for another 18-20 minutes

2. Chop eggplants and sprinkle with salt

3. Add eggplants, tomatoes and the rest of ingredients

4. Cook for another 20-30 minutes or until eggplant is soft

5. When ready remove and serve

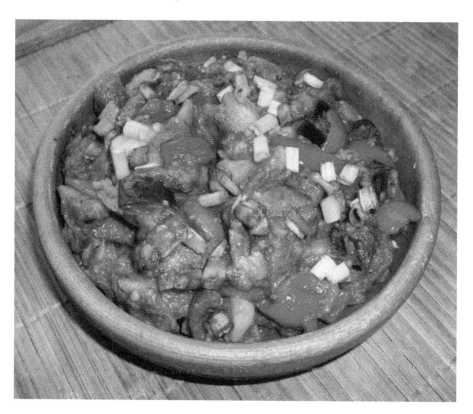

NOODLE SOUP

Serves: *4*

Prep Time: *10*   Minutes

Cook Time: *90*   Minutes

Total Time: *100* Minutes

INGREDIENTS

-       1 chicken

-       1 onion

-       2 carrots

-       2 stalks celery

-       ½ cup spaghetti squash

DIRECTIONS

1. Place a pot over medium heat, add the chicken and cover with water

2. Cook for 50-60 minutes, add onion, celery, carrots and cook for another 30 minutes or until vegetables are soft

3. When ready, remove meat from the chicken bones

4. Pour soup in a bowl

5. Add ½ cup of spaghetti squash noodles to a bowl

6. Season with salt, pepper and serve

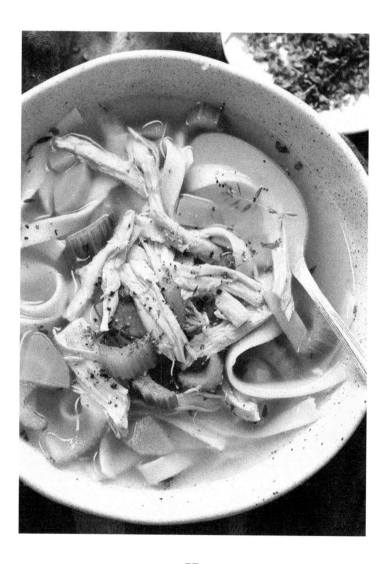

GREEN PESTO PASTA

Serves: *2*

Prep Time: *5*   Minutes

Cook Time: *15*   Minutes

Total Time: *20*   Minutes

INGREDIENTS

- 4 oz. spaghetti

- 2 cups basil leaves

- 2 garlic cloves

- ¼ cup olive oil

- 2 tablespoons parmesan cheese

- ½ tsp black pepper

DIRECTIONS

1. Bring water to a boil and add pasta

2. In a blend add parmesan cheese, basil leaves, garlic and blend

3. Add olive oil, pepper and blend again

4. Pour pesto onto pasta and serve when ready

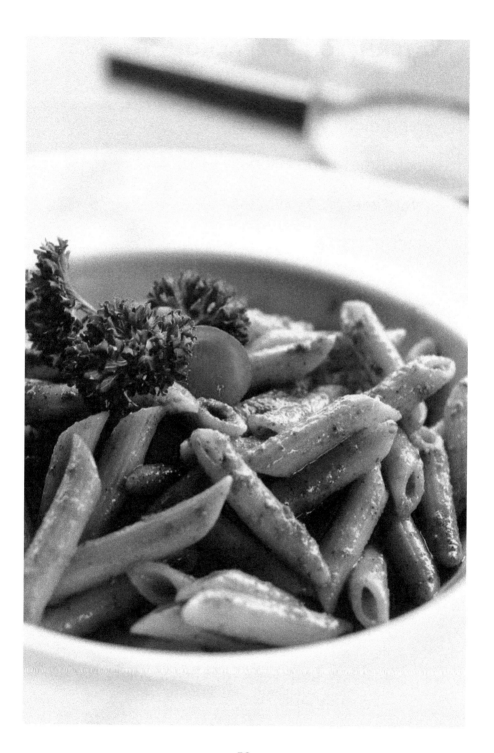

WATERMELON GAZPACHO

Serves: *3*

Prep Time: *10* Minutes

Cook Time: *10* Minutes

Total Time: *20* Minutes

INGREDIENTS

- 2 cups ripe watermelon

- 1 red pepper

- ¼ onion

- 3 tablespoons red wine vinegar

- 6 tablespoons cranberry juice

- Italian basil leaves as needed

DIRECTIONS

1. Puree all ingredients, except the basil, until smooth

2. Refrigerate to chill

3. Serve garnished with basil, onion, tomato or cucumber

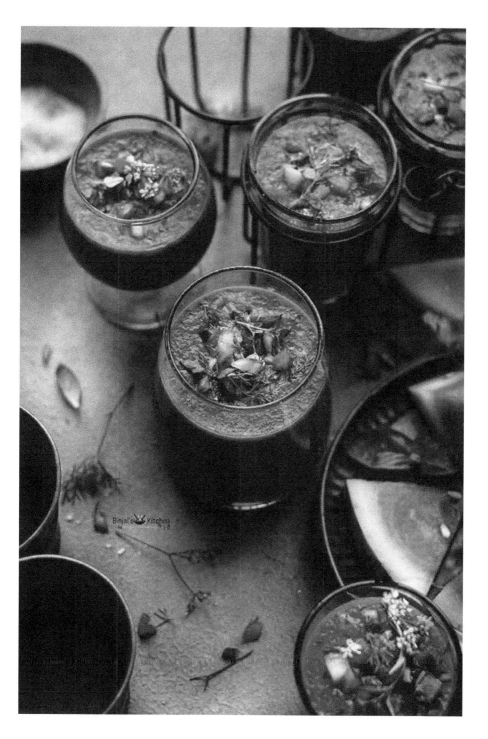

ZUCCHINI CIOPPINO

Serves: *4*

Prep Time: *10* Minutes

Cook Time: *35* Minutes

Total Time: *45* Minutes

INGREDIENTS

- 1 cup water

- 1 zucchini

- 4 tomatoes

- black pepper to taste

- ¼ red onion

- ¼ tsp garlic

- 1 bag frozen seafood blend

- 2 tablespoons apple cider vinegar

DIRECTIONS

1. In a pot add water, zucchini and cook on high heat for 12-15 minutes

2. Add tomatoes, onion, garlic, black pepper, frozen seafood, and cover

3. Add 2 tablespoons of vinegar and cook for another 15-18 minutes

4. When ready remove from heat and serve with lemon juice or lemon wedges

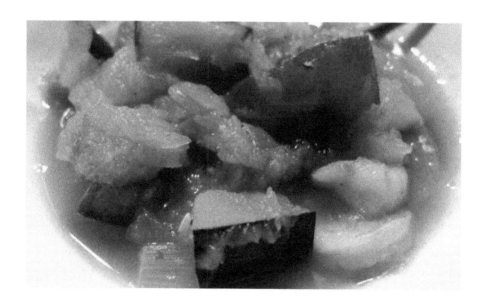

SHREDDED NAPA CABBAGE

Serves: *4*

Prep Time: *5*   Minutes

Cook Time: *50*   Minutes

Total Time: *55*   Minutes

INGREDIENTS

-       1 tablespoon butter

-       1 onion

-       1 green bell pepper

-       2 stalks celery

-       1 lb. ground beef

-        1 cup tomatoes

-       ¼ tsp garlic

-       1 bay leaf

-       1 tsp oregano

-       1 tsp paprika

-       ¼ tsp red pepper flakes

DIRECTIONS

1. In a pot sauté pepper, onion, and celery for 6-8 minutes

2. Add beef, tomatoes and stir to combine

3. Bring to a boil and cook for 50-60 minutes or until liquid has evaporated

4. Serve over napa cabbage

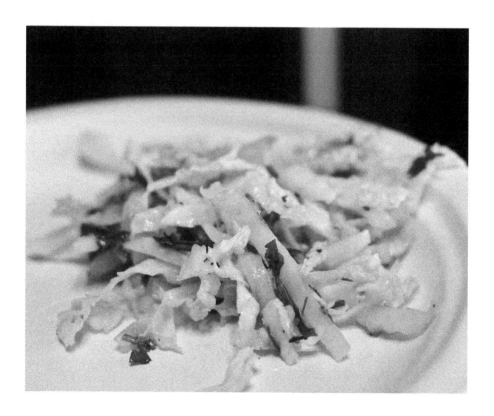

PUMPKIN PANCAKES

Serves: *4*

Prep Time: *5*   Minutes

Cook Time: *15*   Minutes

Total Time: *20*   Minutes

INGREDIENTS

- 1 egg

- ¼ cup pumpkin puree

- 1 tablespoon honey

- ¼ cup almond flour

- ¼ tsp pumpkin pie spice

- ¼ tsp vanilla extract

- ¼ tsp baking soda

DIRECTIONS

1. In a bowl stir in honey, pumpkin and beaten egg

2. Add salt, vanilla, almond flour, spice, and baking soda, stir to combine

3. In a skillet pour ¼ batter and cook for 2-3 minutes per side

4. When ready remove and serve with honey

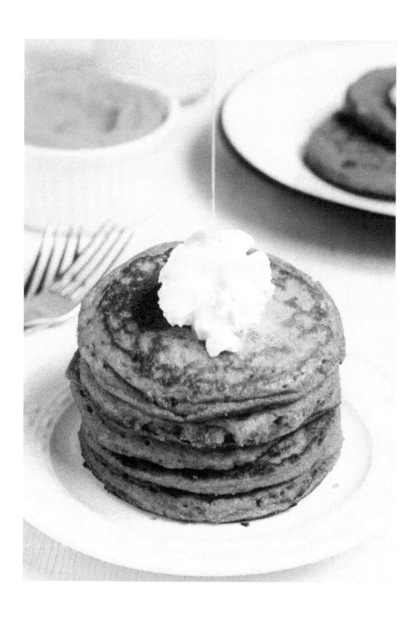

TURKEY & VEGGIES STUFFED PEPPERS

Serves: *4*

Prep Time: *10*   Minutes

Cook Time: *40*   Minutes

Total Time: *50*   Minutes

INGREDIENTS

- 4 red bell peppers

- 1 lb. ground turkey

- 1 tablespoon olive oil

- ¼ onion

- 1 cup mushrooms

- 1 zucchini

- ½ green bell pepper

- ½ yellow bell pepper

- 1 cup spinach

- 1 tsp Italian seasoning

- ¼ tsp garlic powder

- 1 pinch of salt

DIRECTIONS

1. Preheat the oven to 325 F

2. In a pot bring water to boil, add pepper and cook for 5-6 minutes

3. In a skillet cook the turkey until brown and set aside

4. In another pan add onion, olive oil, mushrooms, zucchini, green, yellow pepper, spinach and cook until tender

5. Add remaining ingredients to the turkey and cook until done

6. Stuff the peppers with the mixture and place them into a casserole dish

7. Bake for 15-18 minutes or until done

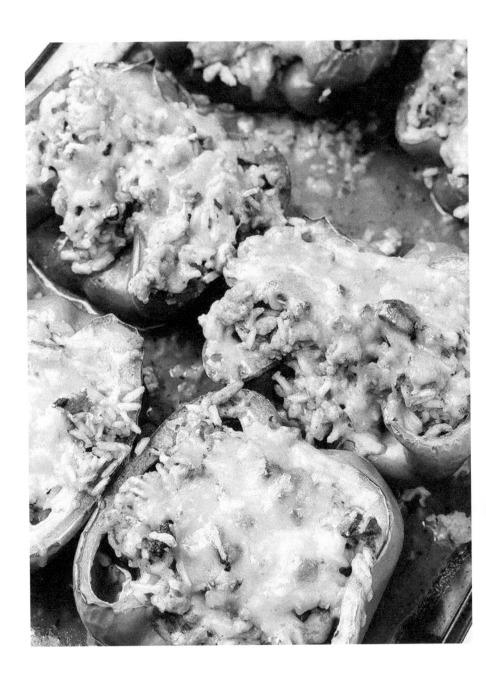

SIMPLE CHOWDER

Serves: 6

Prep Time: *10* Minutes

Cook Time: *50* Minutes

Total Time: *60* Minutes

INGREDIENTS

- ¼ tablespoon butter

- ¼ onion

- 2 carrots

- 2 stalks celery

- 2 cups cauliflower florets

- ¼ cup coconut milk

- 1 cup water

- 1 cup tuna

- juice of ½ lime

- ¼ tsp cilantro

- salt to taste

- pepper to taste

DIRECTIONS

1. In a saucepan sauté carrot, onion, and celery for 4-5 minutes

2. Add cauliflower, water, coconut milk and bring to a boil

3. Reduce heat and simmer for 25-30 minutes

4. Puree 1 cup of soup and bring back to the soup

5. Add lime juice, spices, tuna, and cilantro

6. Stir to combine and cook for another 6-8 minutes

7. When ready remove and serve

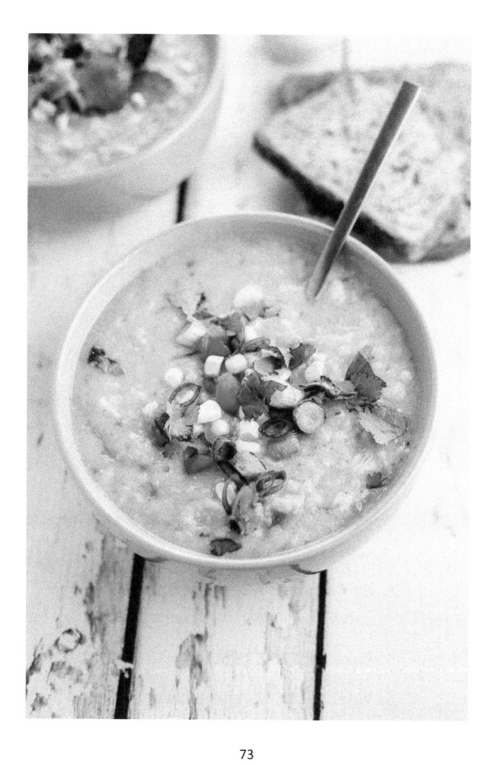

KALE CHIPS

Serves: 6

Prep Time: 10   Minutes

Cook Time: 25   Minutes

Total Time: 35   Minutes

INGREDIENTS

-        1 bunch of kale

-        1 tablespoon olive oil

-        1 tsp salt

DIRECTIONS

1. Preheat the oven to 325 F

2. Chop the kale into chip size pieces

3. Put pieces into a bowl tops with olive oil and salt

4. Spread the leaves in a single layer onto a parchment paper

5. Bake for 20-25 minutes

6. When ready, remove and serve

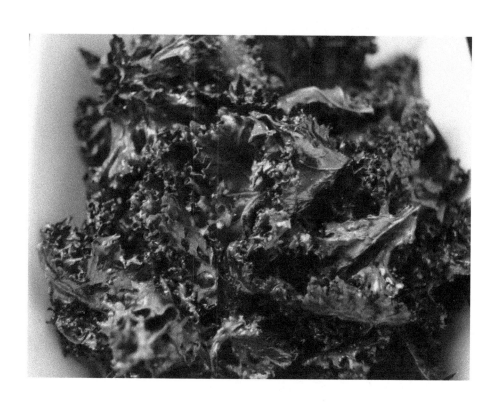

ROASTED BUTTERNUT SQUASH

Serves: *4*

Prep Time: *10* Minutes

Cook Time: *35* Minutes

Total Time: *45* Minutes

INGREDIENTS

-        2 lbs. butternut squash

-        2 carrots

-        1 onion

-        ¼ tsp salt

-        ½ tsp sage

-        ½ dried thyme

-        ¼ tsp marjoram

-        2 tablespoons ghee

DIRECTIONS

1. Cut the butternut squash into cubes

2. In a bowl combine ghee with seasoning and pour over vegetables and toss well

3. Cook at 375 F for 30-35

4. When ready remove and serve

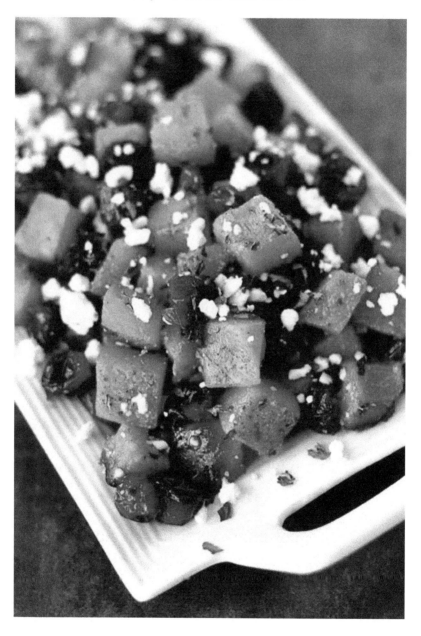

MASHED CAULIFLOWER

Serves: 6

Prep Time: 10 Minutes

Cook Time: 30 Minutes

Total Time: 40 Minutes

INGREDIENTS

- 1 tablespoon butter

- 4 garlic cloves

- 1 head cauliflower

- 2 tablespoons butter

- 1 tsp salt

DIRECTIONS

1. Preheat the skillet to 400 F

2. In a baking dish combine garlic cloves with butter, roast for 12-15 minutes

3. In a pot bring water to boil, add chopped cauliflower and cook for 12-15 minutes

4. Place roasted garlic, 2 tablespoons butter and cauliflower in a blender and blend until smooth

5. When ready remove and serve

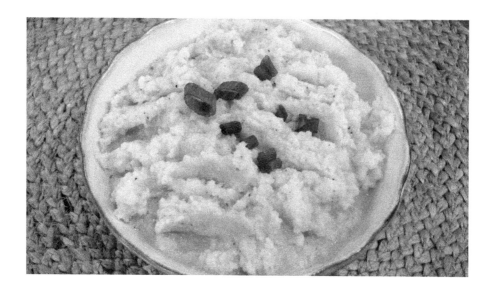

CAULIFLOWER WINGS

Serves: *4*

Prep Time: *10*   Minutes

Cook Time: *50*   Minutes

Total Time: *60*   Minutes

INGREDIENTS

- 1 head cauliflower

- ¼ unsweetened almond milk

- ¼ cup water

- 1 tsp garlic powder

- 1 tsp onion powder

- 1 tsp cumin

- 1 tsp paprika

- ½ tsp salt

- ¼ tsp ground pepper

VINEGAR SAUCE

- 1 tablespoon vegan butter

-        2 tablespoons apple cider vinegar (SCD Safe vinegar)

-        1 tablespoon water

-        1 pinch of salt

DIRECTIONS

1. Preheat the oven to 425 F

2. Mix all wing ingredients in a bowl and submerge each cauliflower floret into the mix

3. Place florets on a prepared baking sheet

4. Bake for 10 minutes, flip and bake for another 10 minutes or until golden brown

5. Remove the cauliflower from the oven and serve with vinegar sauce

6. When ready season with pepper and salt and serve

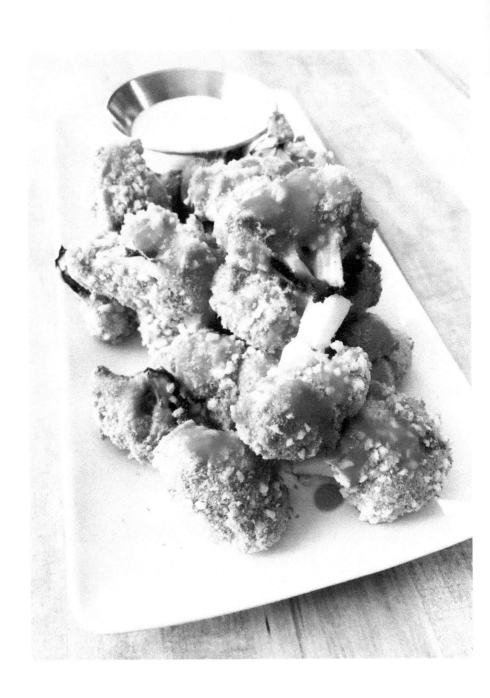

BRUSSEL SPROUTS AND PEAR

Serves: *4*

Prep Time: *5*   Minutes

Cook Time: *15*   Minutes

Total Time: *20*   Minutes

INGREDIENTS

- 2 lb. Brussel sprouts

- ¼ cup chicken broth

- 6 oz. sugar-free bacon

- 2 pears

- salt to taste

DIRECTIONS

1. In a skillet cook the bacon until crispy, remove and set aside

2. Add Brussel sprouts, broth and cook until tender

3. Add the pears, bacon, salt and cook until tender

4. When ready remove and serve

83

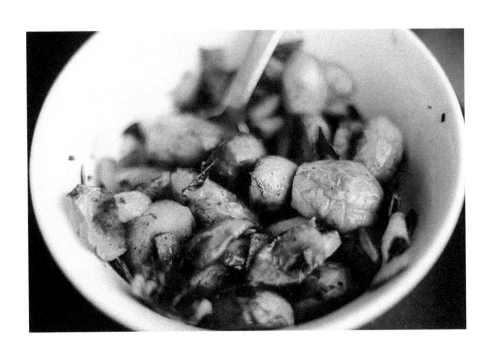

ROASTED VEGETABLES

Serves: *12*

Prep Time: *10* Minutes

Cook Time: *120* Minutes

Total Time: *130* Minutes

INGREDIENTS

- 1 lb. carrots

- 1 lb. green beans

- 1 red onion

- 1 yellow pepper

- 1 orange

- 3 garlic cloves

- 2 tablespoons ghee

- 5 spring thyme

- 1 tsp salt

- ¼ tsp pepper

- 1 tsp basil

- ¼ tsp paprika

DIRECTIONS

1. Preheat the oven at 425 F

2. In a bowl combine all vegetables together

3. In another bowl combine garlic, basil, paprika, salt, ghee and pepper

4. Pour mixture over vegetables and toss to coat

5. Roast for 18-20 minutes, flip and roast for another 15-18 minutes

6. When ready, remove and serve

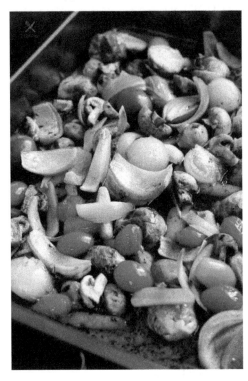

CRANBERRY SALAD

Serves: 2

Prep Time: 5 Minutes

Cook Time: 15 Minutes

Total Time: 20 Minutes

INGREDIENTS

- ½ cup celery

- 1 packet Knox Gelatin

- 1 cup cranberry juice

- 1 can berry cranberry sauce

- 1 cup sour cream

DIRECTIONS

1. In a pan add juice, gelatin, cranberry sauce and cook on low heat

2. Add sour cream, celery and continue to cook

3. Pour mixture into a pan

4. Serve when ready

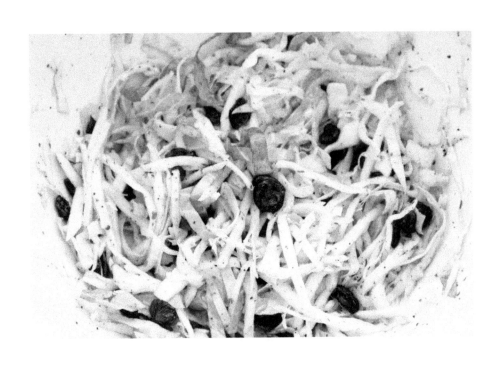

BRUSSELS SPROUT SALAD

Serves: 2

Prep Time: 5 Minutes

Cook Time: 5 Minutes

Total Time: 10 Minutes

INGREDIENTS

- 1 tablespoon olive oil

- 1 cup shallots

- ½ cup celery

- 1 clove garlic

- 6-8 brussels sprouts

- 1 tablespoon thyme leaves

- herbs

DIRECTIONS

1. In a bowl combinie all ingredients together and mix well

2. Serve with dressing

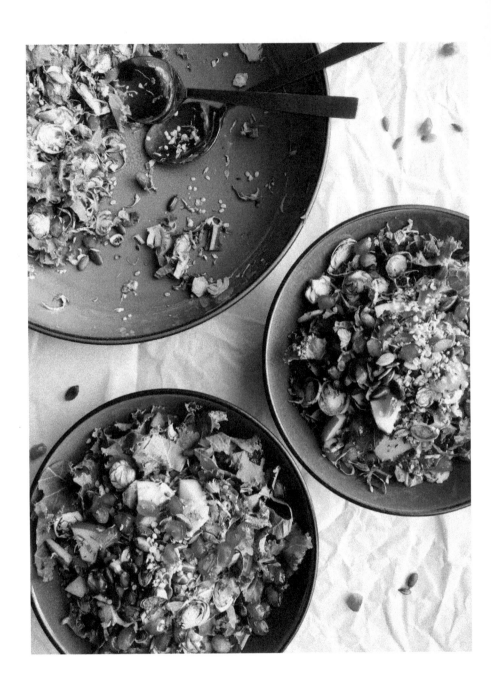

PEARS SALAD

Serves: *2*

Prep Time: *5*   Minutes

Cook Time: *5*   Minutes

Total Time: *10*   Minutes

INGREDIENTS

- ¼ cup almonds

- 4 oz. goat cheese

- 4 cups salad greens

- 1 tablespoon olive oil

- 2-3 pears

- 2 tablespoons honey

DIRECTIONS

1. In a bowl combinie all ingredients together and mix well

2. Serve with dressing

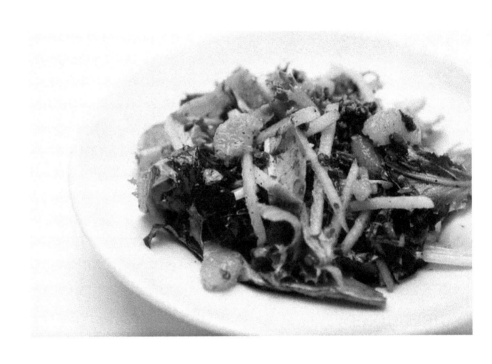

CALIFORNIA SALAD

Serves: 2

Prep Time: 5 Minutes

Cook Time: 5 Minutes

Total Time: 10 Minutes

INGREDIENTS

- 2-3 cups broccoli slaw

- 1-2 bunches green onion

- 1 tablespoon olive oil

- 1 package cooked noodles

- salad dressing

DIRECTIONS

1. In a bowl combinie all ingredients together and mix well

2. Serve with dressing

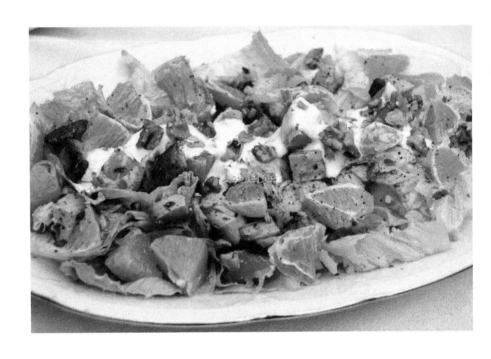

QUINOA SALAD

Serves: *2*

Prep Time: *5*   Minutes

Cook Time: *5*   Minutes

Total Time: *10*   Minutes

INGREDIENTS

-        1 cup cooked quinoa

-        1 handful of spinach leaves

-        1 pear

-        ¼ cup black beans

-        ¼ cup bell pepper

-        ¼ cup cucumber

-        ¼ cup zucchini

DIRECTIONS

1. In a bowl combinie all ingredients together and mix well

2. Serve with dressing

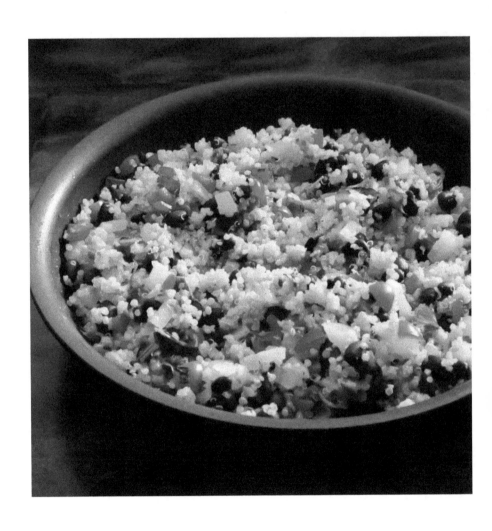

APPLE SLAW

Serves: 2

Prep Time: 5 Minutes

Cook Time: 5 Minutes

Total Time: 10 Minutes

INGREDIENTS

- 4 cups cabbage

- 2 cups apples

- ¼ cup Greek Yogurt

- 2 tablespoons honey

- ¼ tsp salt

DIRECTIONS

1. In a bowl combinie all ingredients together and mix well

2. Serve with dressing

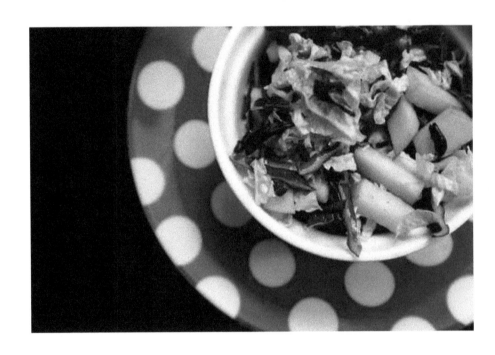

EGG SALAD

Serves: *2*

Prep Time: *5*   Minutes

Cook Time: *5*   Minutes

Total Time: *10*   Minutes

INGREDIENTS

-        3 hard-boiled eggs

-        1 tablespoon tahini

-        ¼ cup olive oil

-        1 garlic clove

-        ½ lb. fava beans

-        2 tomatoes

-        1 cucumber

-        pinch of smoked paprika

DIRECTIONS

1. In a bowl combinie all ingredients together and mix well

2. Serve with dressing

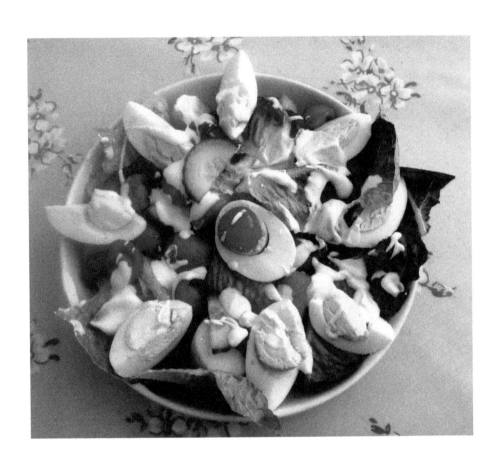

SALMON PASTA SALAD

Serves: 2

Prep Time: 5 Minutes

Cook Time: 5 Minutes

Total Time: 10 Minutes

INGREDIENTS

- 3 oz. cooked penne pasta

- 1 tablespoon olive oil

- 2 cooked salmon fillets

- ¼ lemon juice

- lemon zest

- 1 shallot

- 1 tablespoon capers

- 7-8 olives

- ¼ cup olive oil

DIRECTIONS

1. In a bowl combinie all ingredients together and mix well

2. Serve with dressing

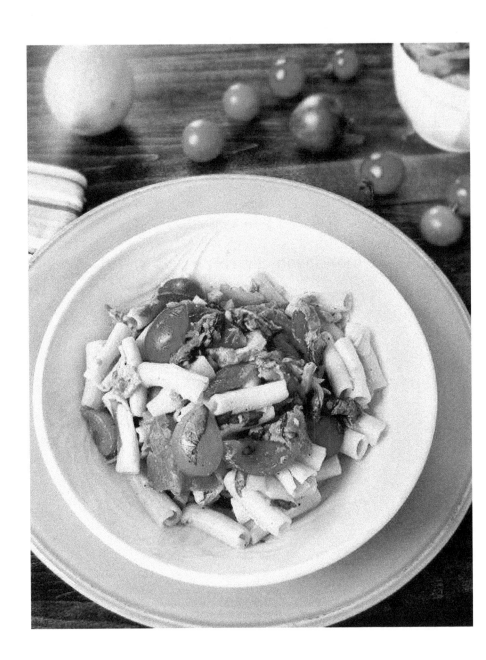

BROCCOLI CASSEROLE

Serves: *4*

Prep Time: *10* Minutes

Cook Time: *15* Minutes

Total Time: *25* Minutes

INGREDIENTS

- 1 onion

- 2 chicken breasts

- 2 tablespoons unsalted butter

- 2 eggs

- 2 cups cooked rice

- 2 cups cheese

- 1 cup parmesan cheese

- 2 cups cooked broccoli

DIRECTIONS

1. Sauté the veggies and set aside

2. Preheat the oven to 425 F

3. Transfer the sautéed veggies to a baking dish, add remaining ingredients to the baking dish

4. Mix well, add seasoning and place the dish in the oven

5. Bake for 12-15 minutes or until slightly brown

6. When ready remove from the oven and serve

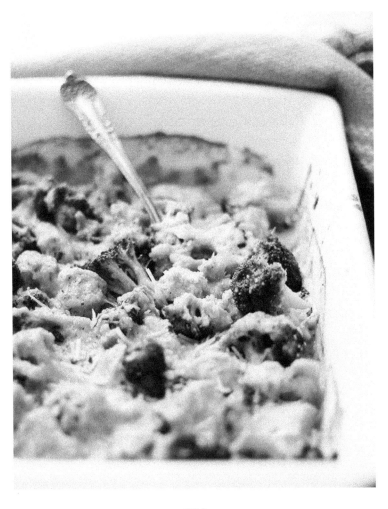

BEAN FRITATTA

Serves: 2

Prep Time: 10 Minutes

Cook Time: 20 Minutes

Total Time: 30 Minutes

INGREDIENTS

- 1 cup black beans

- 1 tablespoon olive oil

- ½ red onion

- 2 eggs

- ¼ tsp salt

- 2 oz. cheddar cheese

- 1 garlic clove

- ¼ tsp dill

DIRECTIONS

1. In a bowl whisk eggs with salt and cheese

2. In a frying pan heat olive oil and pour egg mixture

3. Add remaining ingredients and mix well

4. Serve when ready

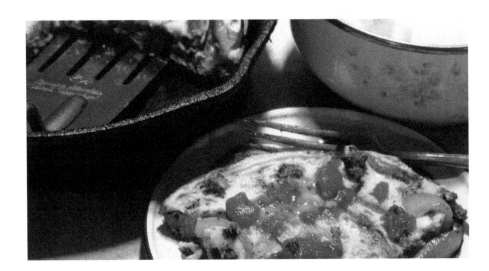

ROASTED SQUASH

Serves: 3-4

Prep Time: 10   Minutes

Cook Time: 20   Minutes

Total Time: 30   Minutes

INGREDIENTS

- 2 delicata squashes

- 2 tablespoons olive oil

- 1 tsp curry powder

- 1 tsp salt

DIRECTIONS

1. Preheat the oven to 400 F

2. Cut everything in half lengthwise

3. Toss everything with olive oil and place onto a prepared baking sheet

4. Roast for 18-20 minutes at 400 F or until golden brown

5. When ready remove from the oven and serve

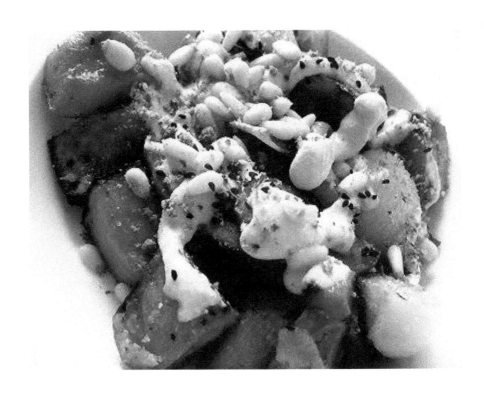

ROASTED FENNEL

Serves: *4*

Prep Time: *10* Minutes

Cook Time: *30* Minutes

Total Time: *40* Minutes

INGREDIENTS

-       4 fennel bulbs

-       1 tablespoon olive oil

-       1 tsp salt

DIRECTIONS

1. Slice the fennel bulb lengthwise into thick slices

2. Drizzle with olive oil and salt

3. Place the fennel bulb into a baking dish

4. Bake at 375 F for 25-30 minutes

5. When ready remove from the oven and serve

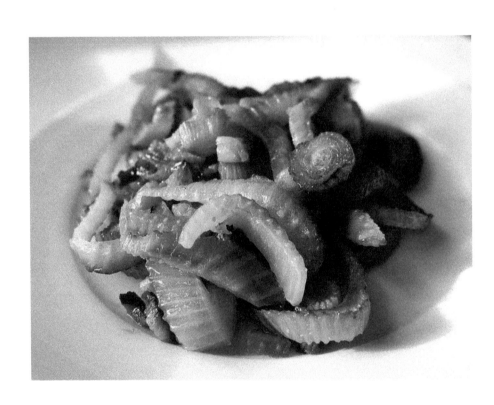